The Best   Pressure Cooker Recipes for Women Over 60

The Ultimate Guide to Easy and Tasty Recipes to Save Time and Impress Your Family and Friends

Elisa D. Fulton

1

Sommario

Introduction

The Ninja Foodi multi-cooker is one of the devices that everyone must have in their cooking area. The gadget can change 4 tiny pieces of equipment: slow cooker, air fryer, pressure cooker as well as dehydrator.

This recipe book consists of a few of the recipes we have actually attempted with the multi-cooker. The recipes vary from breakfast, side dishes, chicken, pork, soups, fish and shellfish, treats, as well as pasta. Additionally, we've put together loads of vegan recipes you ought to attempt. We created these dishes considering newbies which's why the food preparation treatment is organized.

Besides, the meals are tasty, appreciate analysis.

Other Ninja Foodi favorites

Easy And Cheesy Asparagus

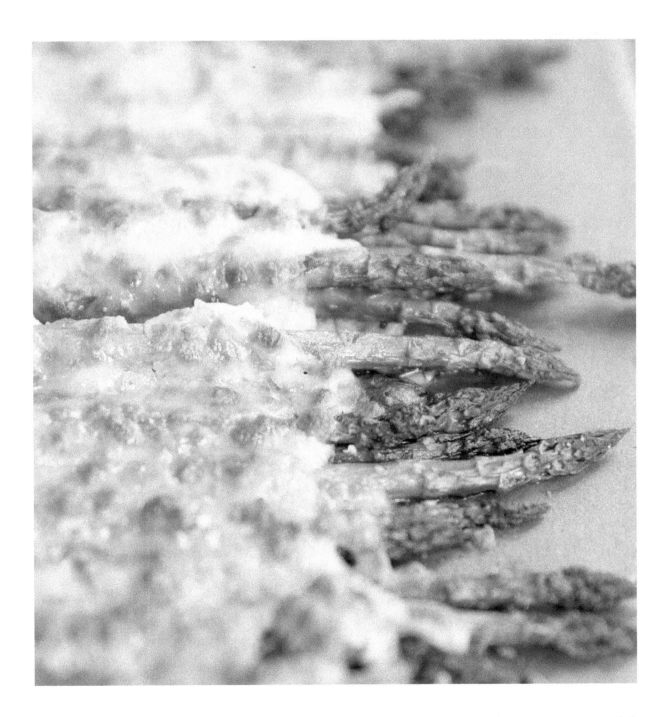

INGREDIENTS (4 Servings)

1 and ½ pounds fresh asparagus ,2 tablespoons olive oil ,4 garlic

cloves, minced

Salt and pepper to taste ,½ cup Colby cheese, shredded

DIRECTIONS (Prep + Cook Time: 13 minutes) Add 1 cup

water to Ninja Foodi. Add steamer basket to Ninja Foodi Place

asparagus and drizzle asparagus with olive oil Scatter garlic over

asparagus. Season with salt and pepper Lock lid and cook on HIGH

pressure for 1 minute. Quick release pressure Serve with cheese

scattered on top. Enjoy!

Creative Srilankan Coconut Dish

INGREDIENTS (4 Servings)

1 tablespoon coconut oil ,1 medium brown onion, halved and

sliced ,1 and ½ teaspoon salt

2 large garlic cloves, diced ,½ a long red chili, sliced ,1 tablespoon

yellow mustard seeds

1 tablespoon turmeric powder ,1 medium cabbage, quartered,

shredded and sliced

1 medium carrot, peeled and sliced ,2 tablespoons lime juice ,½

cup desiccated unsweetened coconut 1 tablespoon olive oil ,1/3

cup water

DIRECTIONS (Prep + Cook Time: 20 minutes) Set your Ninja

Foodi to Saute mode and add coconut oil, once the oil is hot and

add onion and half of the salt. Saute for 3-4 minutes Add garlic,

chili, and spices and Saute for 30 seconds Add cabbage, lime juice,

carrots, coconut, and olive oil and stir well. Add water and stir Lock

up the lid and cook on HIGH pressure for 5 minutes Release the

pressure naturally over 5 minutes followed by a quick

release Serve as a side with chicken/fish. Enjoy!

Quick And Easy Garlic Turkey Breasts

INGREDIENTS (4 Servings)

½ teaspoon garlic powder ,4 tablespoons butter ,¼ teaspoon

dried oregano

1 pound turkey breasts, boneless ,1 teaspoon black pepper ,½

teaspoon salt ,¼ teaspoon dried salt

DIRECTIONS (Prep + Cook Time:20 minutes) Season both

turkey on both sides with garlic powder, dried oregano, dried basil,

salt, and pepper. Set your pot to Saute mode and add breasts and butter. Saute for 2 minutes Lock lid and BAKE/ROAST for 15

minutes at 355 degrees F. Serve and enjoy!

Magnificent Cauliflower Alfredo Zoodles

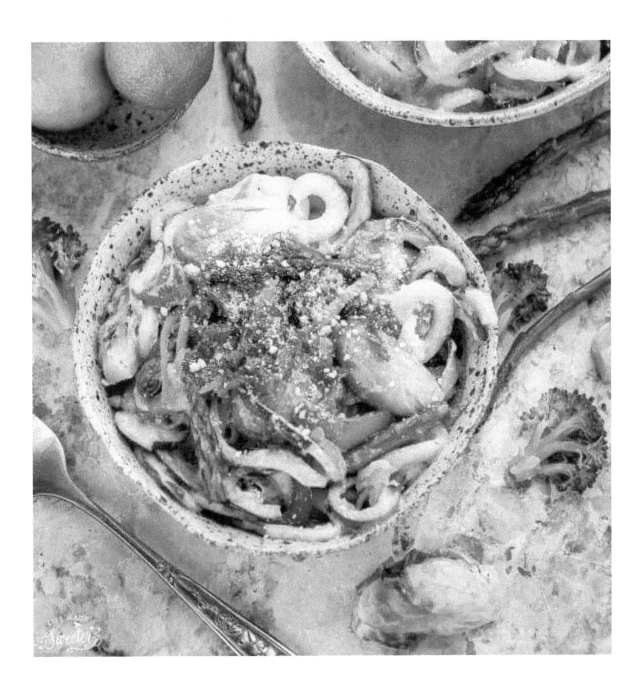

INGREDIENTS (4 Servings)

2 tablespoons butter ,2 garlic cloves ,7-8 cauliflower florets ,1 cup broth 2 teaspoons salt ,2 cups spinach, coarsely chopped

2 green onions, chopped ,1 pound zoodles ,Chopped sundried tomatoes, balsamic vinegar, and cheese for garnish

DIRECTIONS (Prep + Cook Time: 18 minutes) Set your Ninja Foodi to Saute mode and add butter, allow the butter to melt Add garlic cloves and Saute for 2 minutes Add cauliflower, broth, salt and lock up the lid and cook on HIGH pressure for 6 minutes Prepare the zoodles. Perform a naturally release over 10 minutes Use an immersion blender to blend the mixture in the pot to a puree Pour the sauce over the zoodles Serve with a garnish of cheese, sun-dried tomatoes and a drizzle of balsamic vinegar.

Enjoy!

Ham And Hollandaise Delight

INGREDIENTS (4 Servings)

2 whole eggs ,2 tablespoons Hollandaise sauce ,2 ham slices, chopped ,1 and ½ cups + 2 tablespoons water

DIRECTIONS (Prep + Cook Time: 15 minutes) Add 1 and ½ cups water to Ninja Foodi. Lower trivet inside Crack eggs into 2 ramekins. Add a tablespoon of water on top Place ramekins in Ninja Foodi trivet and lock lid, cook on STEAM mode for 2-3 minutes Quick release pressure and top with ham and hollandaise sauce. Serve and enjoy!

Fancy Holiday Lemon Custard

INGREDIENTS (4 Servings)

5 egg yolks ¼ cup fresh squeezed lemon juice ,1 tablespoon

lemon zest ,1 teaspoon pure vanilla extract

1/3 teaspoon liquid stevia ,2 cups heavy cream 1 cup whipped

coconut cream

DIRECTIONS (PREP + COOK TIME: 30 MINUTES) Take a

medium sized bowl and whisk in yolks, lemon juice, zest, vanilla,

and liquid stevia Whisk in heavy cream, divide the mixture

between 4 ramekins Place the included rack in your Ninja Foodi and place ramekins in the rack Add just enough water to reach

halfway to the sides of the ramekins Lock lid and cook on HIGH

pressure for 20 minutes. Release pressure naturally over 10

minutes Remove ramekins and let them cool down Chill in fridge,

top with whipped coconut cream and enjoy!

Generous Gluten Free Pancakes

INGREDIENTS (4 Servings)

1/3 cup almond flour ,½ cup of water ,½ teaspoon chili powder ,1 Serrano pepper, minced

4 tablespoons coconut oil ,3 tablespoons coconut cream ,¼ teaspoon turmeric powder

1 handful cilantro, chopped 6 large eggs ,1 teaspoon salt ,¼ teaspoon pepper ,½ inch ginger, grated ,½ red onion, chopped

DIRECTIONS (PREP + COOK TIME: 26 MINUTES) Take a bowl and add coconut milk, almond flour, spices, and blend well Stir in ginger, Serrano, cilantro, red onion and mix Grease interior of

Ninja Foodi with coconut oil, pour batter in pot and Lock lid, cook

on LOW pressure for 30 minutes. Release pressure naturally over

10 minutes Remove pancake to a platter and serve. Enjoy!

A Wedding Worthy Coconut Cake

INGREDIENTS (4 Servings)

Dry Ingredients , 1 cup almond flour ,½ cup unsweetened shredded coconut

1/3 cup Truvia ,1 teaspoon of apple pie spice ,1 teaspoon of baking powder ,Wet Ingredients ,¼ cup melted butter

2 lightly whisked eggs ,½ cup heavy whipping cream

DIRECTIONS (PREP + COOK TIME: 20 MINUTES) Add all dry ingredients in a bowl and add the wet ingredients one at a time, making sure to gently stir after each addition. Empty batter into a pan and cover with foil Add water 1-2 cups of water to Ninja Foodi,

place steamer rack Place pan in a steamer rack and lock lid. Cook

on HIGH pressure for 40 minutes Naturally, release pressure over

10 minutes. Quick release pressure Remove pan and let it cool for

15-20 minutes. Flip it over onto a platter and garnish as needed.

Serve and enjoy!

Quick Lava Molten Cake For Keto Lovers

INGREDIENTS (4 Servings)

1 whole egg ,2 tablespoons extra virgin olive oil ,3 tablespoons

stevia ,4 tablespoons coconut milk

4 tablespoons all-purpose almond flour ,1 tablespoon cacao

powder ,Pinch of salt Butter for grease

DIRECTIONS (Prep + Cook Time: 20 minutes) Take a ramekin

and grease it up with clarified butter Add 1 cup of water to your

Ninja Foodi. Place a steamer rack or trivet on top of your pot Take

an e medium sized bowl and add all of the listed ingredients, mix them well until you have a nice batter. Transfer the batter to your

ramekins Transfer the ramekins to the steamer rack and lock up

the lid Cook on HIGH pressure for 6 minutes Allow the pressure

to release naturally over 10 minutes and take the cake out. Serve

and enjoy!

A Christmas-y Pot De Crème

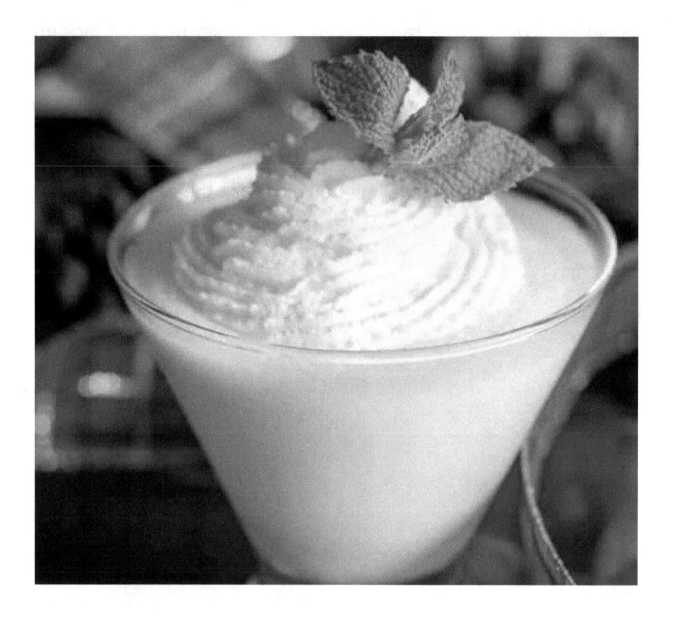

INGREDIENTS (8 Servings)

6 egg yolks 2 cups heavy whipping cream ,½ cup of cocoa

powder 1 tablespoon pure vanilla extract

½ teaspoon stevia Whipped coconut cream for garnish ,Shaved

dark chocolate for garnish

DIRECTIONS (Prep + Cook Time: 3 hours and 10 minutes)

Take a medium sized bowl and whisk in yolks, heavy cream, cocoa

powder, vanilla, stevia Pour mix into 1 and ½ quart baking dish

and place dish in the insert of your Ninja Foodi Add just enough

water until it reaches halfway up the sides of the baking dish Lock

lid and cook on SLOW COOK MODE (LOW) for 3 hours Remove

baking dish and let it cool Chill the dessert completely and garnish

with whipped coconut cream and shaved dark chocolate. Enjoy!

Italian Dark Kale Crisps

INGREDIENTS (4 Servings)

2 cups kale, Italian dark-leaf, 1 teaspoon yeast , 2 tablespoons coconut oil ,½ teaspoon chili flakes ,¼ teaspoon salt

DIRECTIONS (Prep + Cook Time:15 minutes) Take a bowl and tear the kale roughly and place it into the bowl Sprinkle the kale with coconut oil, yeast, chili flakes and salt Mix up the kale well till it becomes consistent Insert the air fryer basket and in the Ninja Foodi and then transfer the kale Air fryer the meal for 10 minutes. Serve and enjoy!

Gentle Keto Butter Fish

INGREDIENTS (6 Servings)

1 pound salmon fillets ,2 tablespoons ginger/garlic paste ,3 green chilies, chopped ,Salt and pepper to taste ,¾ cup butter

DIRECTIONS (Prep + Cook Time: 40 minutes) Season salmon fillets with ginger, garlic paste, salt, pepper Place salmon fillets to Ninja Foodi and top with green chilies and butter Lock lid and BAKE/ROAST for 30 minutes at 360 degrees F Bake for 30 minutes and enjoy!

Slightly Zesty Lamb Chops

INGREDIENTS (4 Servings)

4 tablespoons butter 3 tablespoons lemon juice ,4 lamb chops,

with bone 2 tablespoons almond flour ,1 cup picante sauce

DIRECTIONS (Prep + Cook Time:45 minutes) Coat chops with

almond flour, keep them on the side Set your Ninja Foodi to Saute

mode and add butter, chops Saute for 2 minutes, add picante

sauce and lemon juice Lock lid and cook on HIGH pressure for 40

minutes. Release naturally and serve, enjoy!

Egg Stuffed Avocado Dish

INGREDIENTS (6 Servings)

½ tablespoon fresh lemon juice 1 medium ripe avocado, peeled,

pitted and chopped ,6 organic eggs, boiled, peeled and cut in half

lengthwise

Salt to taste ,½ cup fresh watercress, trimmed

DIRECTIONS (Prep + Cook Time: 15 minutes) Place steamer

basket at the bottom of your Ninja Foodie. Add water Add

watercress on the basket and lock lid Cook on HIGH pressure for

3   minutes,   quick   release   the   pressure   and   drain   the

watercress Remove egg yolks and transfer them to a bowl Add

watercress, avocado, lemon juice, salt into the bowl and mash with

a fork Place egg whites in a serving bowl and fill them with the

watercress and avocado dish Serve and enjoy!

Favorite Peanut Butter Cups

INGREDIENTS (4 Servings)

1 cup butter ,¼ cup heavy cream ,2 ounces unsweetened chocolate ,¼ cup peanut butter, separated ,4 packs stevia

DIRECTIONS (Prep + Cook Time: 35 minutes) Melt peanut butter, butter in a bowl and mix, stir in chocolate, stevia, heavy cream Mix well and pour in baking mold Put mold in Ninja Foodi and lock lid, BAKE/ROAST for 30 minutes at 360 degrees F Transfer to transfer plate and serve. Enjoy!

Simple Veggie And Bacon Platter

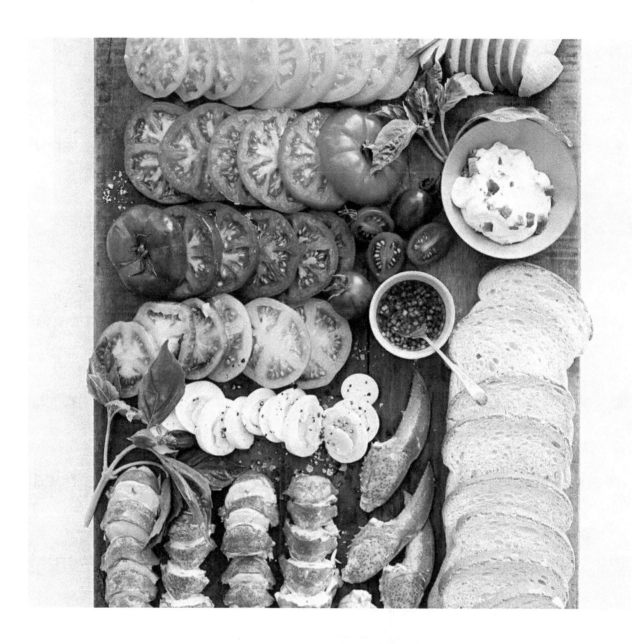

INGREDIENTS (4 Servings)

1 green bell pepper, seeded and chopped ,4 bacon slices ,½ cup

parmesan cheese ,1 tablespoon avocado mayonnaise ,2 scallions,

chopped

DIRECTIONS (Prep + Cook Time: 35 minutes) Arrange bacon

slices in Ninja Foodi, top with avocado mayo, pepper, scallions,

cheese Lock lid and Cook on "BAKE/ROAST" mode for 25 minutes

at 365 degrees F Remove from Foodi and serve, enjoy!

Divine Keto Nut Porridge

INGREDIENTS (4 Servings)

4 teaspoons coconut oil, melted ,1 cup pecans, halved ,2 cups of water ,2 tablespoons stevia ,1 cup cashew nuts, raw and unsalted

DIRECTIONS (Prep + Cook Time: 20 minutes)

Add cashews and pecans to a food processor, pulse until chunky Add nuts mix to Ninja Foodi, stir in water, coconut oil, and stevia Set your pot to Saute mode and cook for 15 minutes. Serve and enjoy!

Quick And Easy Buttery Pancake

INGREDIENTS (4 Servings)

2 cups cream cheese ,2 cups almond flour ,6 large whole

eggs ,1/4 teaspoon salt ,2 tablespoons butter

¼ teaspoon ground ginger ,½ teaspoon cinnamon powder

DIRECTIONS (Prep + Cook Time: 15 minutes) Take a large

bowl and add cream cheese, eggs, 1 tablespoon butter. Blend on

high until creamy. Slow add flour and keep beating. Add salt,

ginger, cinnamon. Keep beating until fully mixed. Set your Ninja

Foodi to Saute mode and grease stainless steel insert. Add butter and heat it up. Add ½ cup batter and cook for 2-3 minutes, flip and

cook the other side Repeat with the remaining batter, Enjoy!

Lovely Bok Choy Soup

INGREDIENTS (4 Servings)

4 chicken thighs ,4 cups beef bone broth ,1 pound Bok choy ,Salt

and pepper to taste ,¼ teaspoon dried dill weed ,1 teaspoon bay

leaf

DIRECTIONS (Prep + Cook Time: 18 minutes) Add chicken

thigh to Ninja Foodi, add 1 cup broth. Lock lid and cook on HIGH

pressure for 8 minutes. Release pressure naturally over 10

minutes. Add remaining ingredients and lock lid again. Cook on

HIGH pressure for 5 minutes more Quick release pressure. Serve

and enjoy!

Flimsy Buffalo Fish

INGREDIENTS (4 Servings)

6 tablespoons butter ,¾ cup Franks red hot sauce ,6 fish fillets ,Salt and pepper to taste ,2 teaspoons garlic powder

DIRECTIONS (Prep + Cook Time: 16 minutes) Set your Ninja Foodi to Saute mode and add butter, fish fillets Saute for 3 minutes and add salt, pepper and garlic powder BAKE/ROAST for 8 minutes at 340 degrees F. Transfer to serving plate and enjoy!

New Broccoli Pops

INGREDIENTS (4 Servings)

1/3 cup parmesan cheese, grated ,2 cups cheddar cheese, grated ,Salt and pepper to taste ,3 eggs, beaten ,3 cups broccoli florets

1 tablespoon olive oil

DIRECTIONS (Prep + Cook Time: 18 minutes) Add broccoli into a food processor and pulse until finely crumbled Transfer broccoli to a large-sized bowl and add remaining ingredients to the bowl, mix well Make small balls using the mixture and let them chill for 30 minutes Place balls in your Ninja Foodi pot and Air

Crisping lid. Let it cook for 12 minutes at 365 degrees F on the "Air

Crisp" mode. Once done, remove and enjoy

Baked Paprika Delight

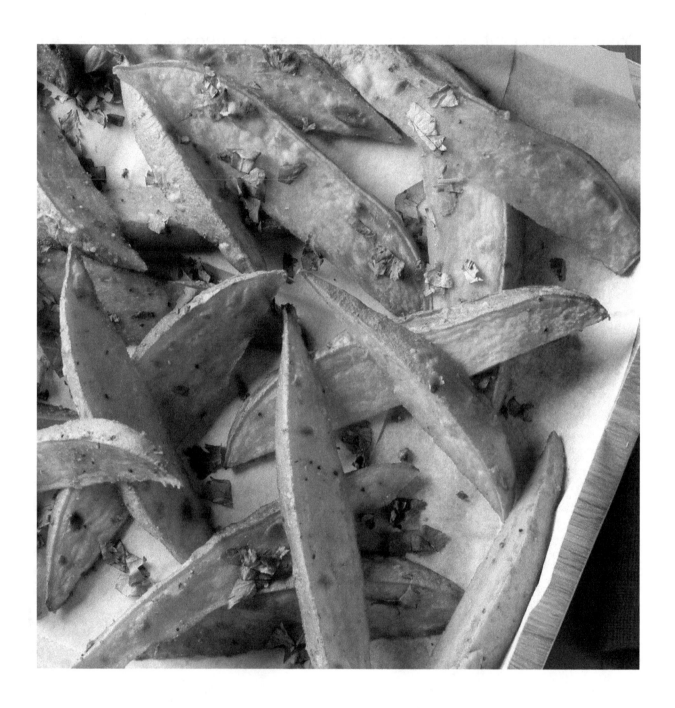

INGREDIENTS (4 Servings)

1 teaspoon smoked paprika ,3 tablespoons butter ,1 pound tiger

shrimps ,Salt, to taste

DIRECTIONS (Prep + Cook Time: 20minutes)

Add listed ingredients in large bowl and marinate shrimps Grease

Ninja Foodi pot with butter and add seasoned shrimps Lock lid and

BAKE/ROAST for 15 minutes at 355 degrees F. Serve and enjoy!

Onion And Tofu Scramble

INGREDIENTS (4 Servings)

4 tablespoons butter ,2 blocks tofu, pressed and cubed into inch

pieces ,Salt and pepper to taste ,1 cup cheddar, grated ,2

medium onions, sliced

DIRECTIONS (Prep + Cook Time: 20 minutes) Take a bowl

and mix in tofu, salt, pepper. Set your Foodi to Saute mode Add

butter and onions, Saute for 3 minutes and add seasoned

tofu Cook for 2 minutes, add Cheddar cheese. Lock lid and cook for 3 minutes on Air Crisp mode at 350 degrees F. Transfer to a

plate, serve and enjoy!

Squash In Sage And Butter Sauce

INGREDIENTS (4 Servings)

1 medium spaghetti squash ,1 and ½ cups of water ,1 bunch fresh

sage ,2 tablespoons olive oil ,1 teaspoon salt ,1/8 teaspoon nutmeg

DIRECTIONS (Prep + Cook Time: 15 minutes) Halve the

squash and scoop out the seeds Add water to your Ninja Foodi and

lower down the squash with the squash halves facing up Stack

them on top of one another. Lock up the lid and cook on HIGH

pressure for 3 minutes Release the pressure over 10

minutes Take a cold Saute pan and add sage, garlic and olive oil and cook on LOW heat, making sure to stir and fry the sage leaves

. Keep it on the side Release the pressure naturally and tease the

squash fibers out from the shell and plop them into the Saute Pan.

Stir well and sprinkle salt and nutmeg. Serve with a bit of cheese

and enjoy!

The Cool Pot-De-Crème

INGREDIENTS (4 Servings)

6 egg yolks ,2 cups heavy whip cream ,1/3 cup cocoa powder ,1 tablespoon pure vanilla extract , ½ teaspoon liquid stevia ,Whipped coconut cream for garnish ,Shaved dark chocolate for garnish

DIRECTIONS (Prep + Cook Time: 30 minutes) Take a medium sized bowl and whisk in yolks, heavy cream, cocoa powder, vanilla and stevia Pour mixture in 1 and ½ quart baking dish, transfer to Nina Foodi insert Add water to reach about half of the ramekin Lock lid and cook on HIGH pressure for 12 minutes, quick

release pressure Remove baking dish from the insert and let it

cool Chill in fridge and serve with a garnish of coconut cream,

shaved chocolate shavings. Enjoy!.

Early Morning Vegetable Stock

INGREDIENTS (4 Servings)

2 small onion, chopped , 2 stocks celery, diced ,2 bay leaves ,2 carrots, diced 1 dried shiitake mushroom , 6 cremini mushrooms, sliced

4 crushed garlic cloves 1 teaspoon whole peppercorn ,2 tablespoons coconut aminos 8 cups cold water ,Dried herbs as needed

DIRECTIONS (Prep + Cook Time: 25 minutes) Prepare the ingredients as mentioned above. Add all of the ingredients to the

Ninja Foodi Lock up the lid and cook on HIGH pressure for 15

minutes Release the pressure naturally over 10 minutes. Strain

the stock through a metal mesh strainer Allow it to cool and chill,

serve!

Heavenly Zucchini Bread

INGREDIENTS (12 Servings)

1 cup almond flour ,2 teaspoons cinnamon ,1/3 cup coconut flour ,½ teaspoon salt ,½ teaspoon baking soda ,1 and ½ teaspoon baking powder

1/3 cup soft coconut oil ,3 whole eggs ,2 teaspoons vanilla bean extract ,1 cup sweetener ,2 cups shredded zucchini ,½ cup pecans, chopped

DIRECTIONS (Prep + Cook Time: 3 hours and 25 minutes)

Take a bowl Add coconut and almond flour, salt, baking soda and powder, cinnamon and xanthan gum. Keep it on the side. Take

another bowl and mix oil, vanilla, eggs, and sugar, mix well Blend

in shredded zucchini and nuts. Pour the baking soda into the bowl

with zucchini and stir well. Pour the mixture into your prepared

pan Place your trivet/rack in your Ninja Foodi and place pan on

top of the trivet Cook on SLOW COOK MODE (HIGH) for 3 hours.

Let it cool and wrap in foil, place in the fridge. Serve and enjoy!

Sensational Carrot Puree

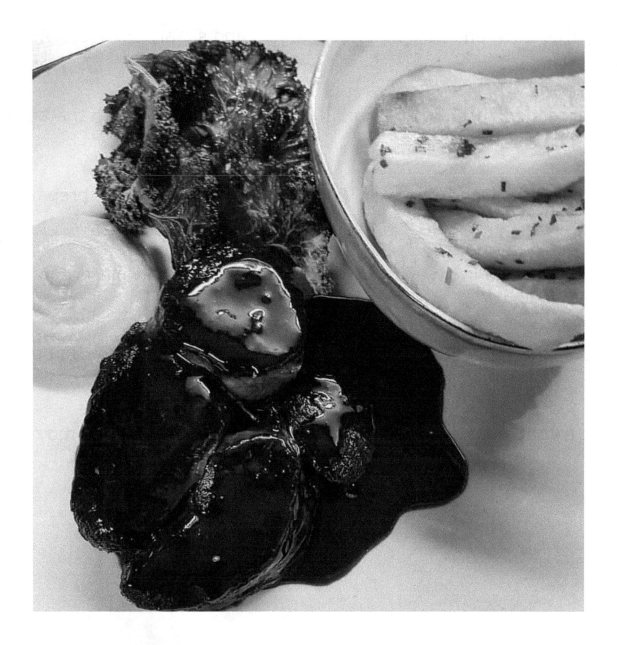

INGREDIENTS (4 Servings)

1 and a ½ pound carrots, chopped ,1 tablespoon of butter at room

temperature ,1 tablespoon of agave nectar ,¼ teaspoon of sea

salt 1 cup of water

DIRECTIONS (Prep + Cook Time: 14 minutes) Clean and peel

your carrots properly. Roughly chop up them into small pieces Add

1 cup of water to your Pot Place the carrots in a steamer basket

and place the basket in the Ninja Foodi Lock up the lid and cook

on HIGH pressure for 4 minutes. Perform a quick release Transfer

the carrots to a deep bowl and use an immersion blender to blend

the carrots Add butter, nectar, salt, and puree. Taste the puree

and season more if needed. Enjoy!

Deserving Mushroom Saute

INGREDIENTS (8 Servings)

1 pound white mushrooms, stems trimmed ,2 tablespoons

unsalted butter ,½ teaspoon salt ,¼ cup of water

DIRECTIONS (Prep + Cook Time: 25 minutes) Quarter

medium mushrooms and cut any large mushrooms into eight Put

mushrooms, butter, and salt in your Foodi's inner pot Add water

and lock pressure lid, making sure to seal the valve Cook on HIGH

pressure for 5 minutes, quick release pressure once did Once

done, set your pot to Saute mode on HIGH mode and bring the mix to a boil over 5 minutes until all the water evaporates Once the

butter/water has evaporated, stir for 1 minute until slightly

browned. Enjoy!

Simple Weeknight Vanilla Yogurt

INGREDIENTS (4 Servings)

½ cup full-fat milk , ¼ cup yogurt started 1 cup heavy cream , ½

tablespoon vanilla extract ,2 teaspoons stevia

DIRECTIONS (Prep + Cook Time: 12 hours and 10 minutes)

Add milk to your Ninja Foodi and stir in heavy cream, vanilla

extract, stevia Stir well, let the yogurt sit for a while. Lock lid and

cook on SLOW COOKER mode for 3 hours Take a small bowl and

add 1 cup milk with the yogurt starter, bring this mixture to the pot Lock lid and wrap Foodi in two small towels. Let it sit for 9

hours (to allow it to culture) Refrigerate and serve. Enjoy!

Spiced Up Jack Cheese Muffin

INGREDIENTS (4 Servings)

¼ cup pepper jack cheese, shredded ,4 bacon slices ,4 whole

eggs ,1 Green onion, chopped ,Pinch of garlic powder ,Pinch of

pepper

¼ teaspoon salt 1 and ½ cups of water

DIRECTIONS (Prep + Cook Time: 20 minutes) Set your Ninja

Foodi to Saute mode and add bacon, cook for a few minutes until

crispy Wipe bacon grease, pour water and lower rack Take a bowl

and beat eggs, pepper, garlic powder, salt. Crumbled bacon and add to the mixture Stir in onion and cheese. Pour mix into 4

silicone muffin cups Arrange on rack and lock lid. Cook on HIGH

for 8 minutes Quick release pressure. Serve and enjoy!

Crispy Tofu And Mushrooms

INGREDIENTS (2Servings)

8 tablespoons parmesan cheese, shredded ,2 cups fresh mushrooms, chopped ,2 blocks tofu, pressed and cubed ,Salt and pepper to taste 8 tablespoons butter

DIRECTIONS (Prep + Cook Time: 20 minutes) Take a bowl and mix in tofu, salt, and pepper Set your Ninja Foodi to Saute mode and add seasoned tofu, Saute for 5 minutes Add mushroom, cheese and Saute for 3 minutes. Lock crisping lid and Air Crisp for 3 minutes at 350 degrees F. Transfer to serving plate and enjoy!

Creamy Beef And Garlic Steak

INGREDIENTS (4 Servings)

½ cup butter ,4 garlic cloves, minced ,2 pounds beef top sirloin steak ,Salt and pepper to taste ,1 and ½ cup cream

DIRECTIONS (Prep + Cook Time: 45 minutes) Rub beef sirloin steaks with garlic, salt, and pepper. Marinate beef with butter, cream and keep it on the side. Place grill in Ninja Foodi and transfer the steaks to the Foodi Lock lid and BROIL for 30 minutes at 365 degrees F, making sure to flip about after halfway through. Serve and enjoy!

Come-Back Cauliflower And Parm

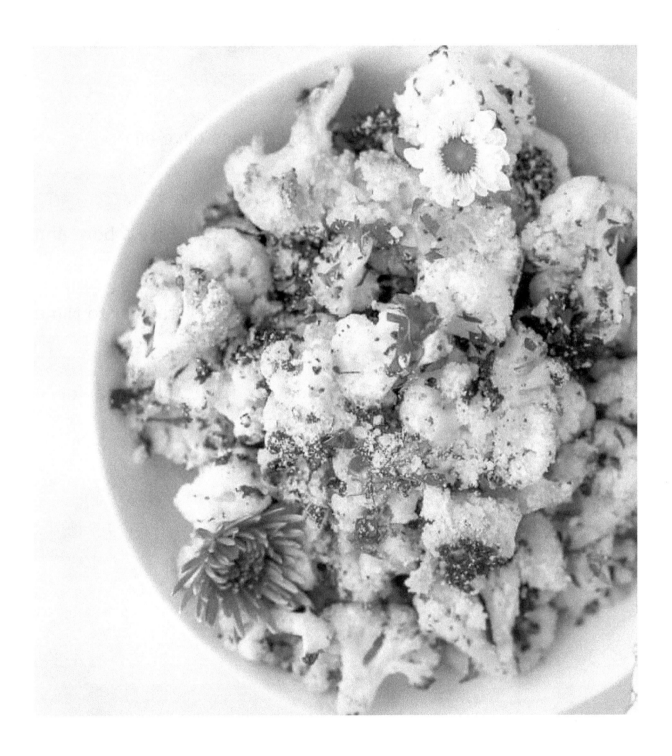

INGREDIENTS (4 Servings)

1 cauliflower head ,½ cup vegetable stock ,2 garlic cloves,

minced ,Salt and pepper to taste ,1/3 cup grated parmesan

1 tablespoons parsley, chopped 3 tablespoons olive oil

DIRECTIONS (Prep + Cook Time: 9 minutes) Take a bowl and

add oil, garlic, salt, pepper cauliflower, and toss. Transfer to Ninja

Foodi Add stock and lock lid, cook on HIGH pressure for 4

minutes Add parsley, parmesan and toss. Serve and enjoy!

Over The Weekend Apple And Sprouts

INGREDIENTS (4 Servings)

1 green apple, julienned ,1 and ½ teaspoon olive oil ,4 cups

alfalfa sprouts ,Salt and pepper to taste ,¼ cup of coconut milk

DIRECTIONS (Prep + Cook Time: 20 minutes) Set your Ninja

Foodi to Saute mode and add oil, let it heat up Add apple, sprouts,

and stir. Lock lid and cook on HIGH pressure for 5 minutes Add

salt, pepper, coconut milk and stir well. Serve3 and enjoy!

Runny Eggs In A Cup

INGREDIENTS (4 Servings)

4 whole eggs ,1 cup mixed veggies, diced ,½ cup cheddar cheese, shredded

¼ cup half and half ,Salt and pepper to taste ,½ cup shredded cheese

DIRECTIONS (Prep + Cook Time:10 minutes) Take a bowl and add eggs, cheese, veggies, half and a half, pepper, salt and chop up cilantro Mix well and divide the mix amongst four ½ a pint wide mouth mason jars (or similar containers). Slightly put the lid on top Add 2 cups of water to your pot and place a steamer rack

on top Place the egg jars on your steamer. Lock up the lid and

cook for 5 minutes at HIGH pressure Quick release the pressure.

Remove the jars and top them up with ½ a cup of cheese Serve

immediately or broil a bit to allow the cheese to melt

The Delightful Cauliflower And Cheese "Cake"

INGREDIENTS (4 Servings)

2 cups cauliflower, riced ,2 tablespoons cream cheese , ½ cup

half and half ,½ cup cheddar cheese, shredded Salt and pepper

to taste

DIRECTIONS (Prep + Cook Time:25 minutes) Take a

heatproof dish and add all of the listed ingredients Cover the dish

with an aluminum foil. Add 1 and a ½ cup of water to your Ninja

Foodi Place a trivet or steamer basket on top. Transfer the covered

trivet on top of your basket Lock up the lid and cook for 5 minutes at HIGH pressure. Allow the pressure to release naturally over 10

minutes Heat up your oven broiler and broil the cauliflowers a bit

and broil them well until the cheese Is brown. Enjoy!

Grandmother's Pumpkin Carrot Cake

INGREDIENTS (4 Servings)

1 tablespoon extra-virgin olive oil , 2 cups carrots, shredded , 2 cups pureed pumpkin , ½ sweet onion, finely chopped ,1 cup heavy whip cream

½ cup cream cheese, soft ,2 whole eggs ,1 tablespoon granulated Erythritol ,1 teaspoon ground nutmeg ½ teaspoon salt ¼ cup pumpkin seeds, garnish ¼ cup of water

DIRECTIONS (Prep + Cook Time: 25 minutes)

1.Add oil to your Ninja Foodi pot and whisk In carrots, pumpkin,

onion, heavy cream, cream cheese, eggs, Erythritol, nutmeg, salt,

and water. Stir and lock lid 2.Cook on HIGH pressure for 10

minutes Release pressure naturally over 10 minutes 3.Serve with

a topping of pumpkin seeds. Enjoy!

Lemon And Ricotta Party-Friendly Cheesecake

INGREDIENTS (4 Servings)

8 ounces cream cheese ,¼ cup Truvia ,1 lemon – zested and juiced ,1/3 cup ricotta cheese ,½ teaspoon lemon extract ,2 whole eggs

For topping Natural sweetener as needed ,1 tablespoon sour cream

DIRECTIONS (Prep + Cook Time: 20 minutes) Take your blender and add all the ingredients except eggs, blend well Add eggs and blend on low speed, making sure to not over beat the eggs Add batter to pan and cover with foil. Add trivet to Ninja

Foodi and 2 cups water Place baking pan in trivet and lock lid, cook

on HIGH pressure for 30 minutes Release pressure naturally over

10 minutes Blend in sweetener and sour cream in a bowl and

decorate the cake with frosting. Enjoy!

Heart Melting Choco-Mousse

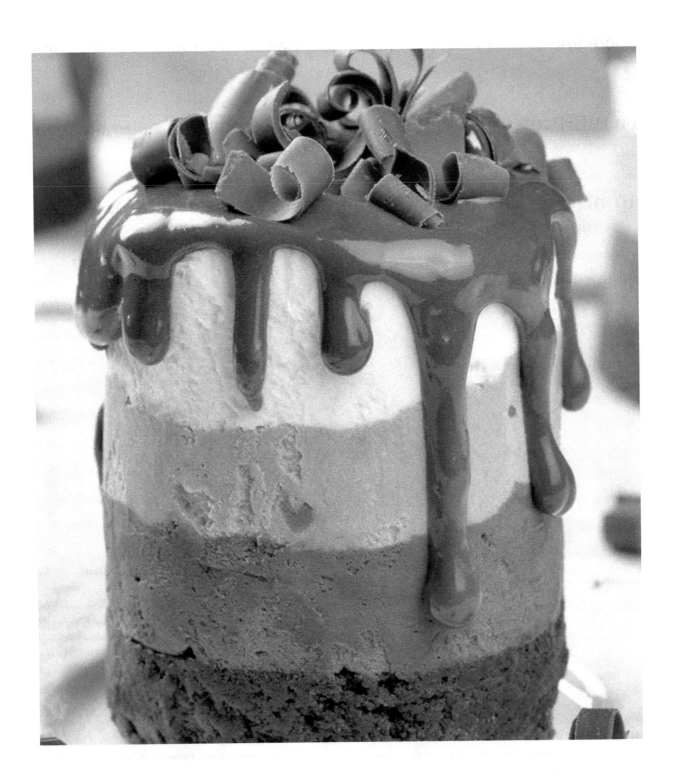

INGREDIENTS (4 Servings)

4 egg yolks ,¼ cup of water ,¼ cup cacao ½ cup Swerve ,½ cup whipping cream ,½ teaspoon vanilla ½ cup almond milk ,¼ teaspoon of sea salt

DIRECTIONS (Prep + Cook Time: 6 hours and 20 minutes)

Take a bowl and whisk in eggs. Add water, swerve, cacao in a saucepan and mix well Stir in milk and cream, let the mixture warm over medium heat until it reaches a boil, remove heat.

Measure 1 tablespoon of chocolate mix into the dish with eggs Whisk and slowly empty the remaining chocolate into the mixture Empty the mousse mix into 5 ramekins. Add 1 and ½ cups water to Instant Pot. Place a trivet Place the trivets into the trivet

and lock lid, cook on HIGH pressure for 6 minutes Quick release

pressure. Chill in the fridge for 6 hours, enjoy!

Quick Ginger And Sesame Chicken

INGREDIENTS (4 Servings)

1 and ½ pounds chicken thighs, no skin , 2 tablespoons coconut

aminos 1 tablespoon agave ,1 tablespoon ginger, minced

1 tablespoon garlic-sesame oil 1 tablespoon rice vinegar ,Red

onion, sliced for salad ,Carrots julienned for salad ,Cucumbers

julienned for salad

DIRECTIONS (Prep + Cook Time:15 minutes) Slice thigh into

large chunks and add rest of the ingredients to a heat-safe

dish Place foil over the bowl. Add 2 cups water to Ninja Foodi Place steamer rack in Ninja Foodi and place the bowl over the rack Lock

lid and cook on HIGH pressure for 10 minutes. Naturally, release

pressure over 10 minutes Shred meat and serve with a tossing of

the salad. Enjoy!

Simple Broccoli Florets

INGREDIENTS (4 Servings)

4 tablespoons butter, melted ,Salt and pepper to taste ,2 pounds

broccoli florets ,1 cup whipping cream

DIRECTIONS (Prep + Cook Time: 16 minutes) Place a

steamer basket in your Ninja Foodi (bottom part) and add

water Place florets on top of the basket and lock lid Cook on HIGH

pressure for 5 minutes. Quick release pressure Transfer florets

from the steamer basket to the pot. Add salt, pepper, butter, and stir Lock crisping lid and cook on Air Crisp mode for 360 degrees

F. Serve and enjoy!

Delicious Creamy Crepes

INGREDIENTS (4 Servings)

1 and ½ teaspoon, Splenda 3 organic eggs ,3 tablespoons

coconut flour ,½ cup heavy cream ,3 tablespoons coconut oil,

melted and divided

DIRECTIONS (Prep + Cook Time: 35 minutes) Take a bowl

and mix in 1 and ½ tablespoons coconut oil, Splenda, eggs, salt

and mix well Beat well until mixed. Add coconut flour and keep

beating. Stir in heavy cream, beat well Set your Ninja Foodi to

Saute mode and add ¼ of the mixture Saute for 2 minutes on each

side. Repeat until all ingredients are used up. Enjoy!

Terrific Baked Spinach Quiche

INGREDIENTS (2 Servings)

1 tablespoons butter, melted ,1 pack frozen spinach, thawed ,5

organic eggs, beaten ,Salt and pepper to taste ,3 cups monetary

jack cheese, shredded

DIRECTIONS (Prep + Cook Time: 20 minutes) Set your pot

to Saute mode and add butter, spinach Saute for 3 minutes,

transfer dish out of the bowl Add eggs, Monterey Jack cheese, salt,

pepper to a bowl and transfer to the greased mold Place molds

inside Ninja Foodi and lock lid, cook on BAKE/ROAST mode for 30 minutes at 360 degrees F. Remove from Ninja Foodi and cut into

wedges. Serve and enjoy!

Nutty Assorted Collection

INGREDIENTS (4 Servings)

1 tablespoon butter, melted , ½ cup raw cashew nuts ,1 cup of raw almonds Salt to taste

DIRECTIONS (Prep + Cook Time: 20 minutes) Add nuts to your Ninja Foodi pot Lock lid and cook on "Air Crisp" mode for 10 minutes at 350 degrees F Remove nuts into a bowl and add melted butter and salt. Toss well to coat Return the mix to your Ninja Foodi, lock lid and bake for 5 minutes on BAKE/ROAST mode Serve and enjoy!

Lovely Yet "Stinky" Garlic

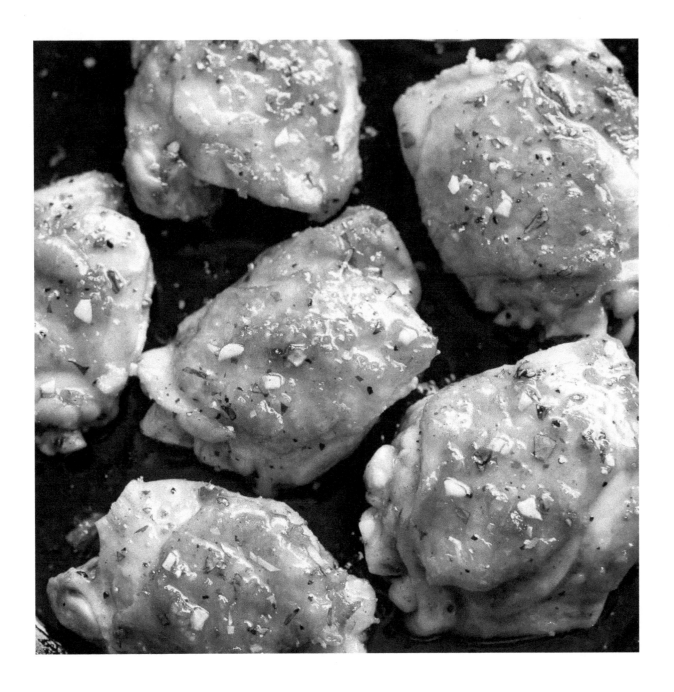

INGREDIENTS (6Servings)

3 large garlic bulb ,A drizzle of olive oil ,1 cup of water

DIRECTIONS (Prep + Cook Time: 20 minutes) Place your

steamer rack on top of the Ninja Foodi. Add 1 cup of water Prepare

the garlic by slicing the top portion Place the bulbs in your steamer

basket and lock up the lid Cook on HIGH pressure for about 6

minutes Allow the pressure to release naturally over 10 minutes.

Take the garlic out using tongs (very hot!) and drizzle olive oil on

top. Broil for about 5 minutes and serve!

Cool "Cooked" Ice Tea

INGREDIENTS (4 Servings)

4 teabags ,6 cups of water ,2 tablespoons agave nectar

DIRECTIONS (Prep + Cook Time: 9 minutes) Add the listed ingredients to your Ninja Foodi and lock up the lid Cook on HIGH pressure for 4 minutes. Release the pressure naturally Allow it to cool and serve over ice. Enjoy!

Juicy Keto Lamb Roast

INGREDIENTS (4 Servings)

2 pounds lamb roast ,1 cup onion soup ,1 cup beef broth ,Salt

and pepper

DIRECTIONS (Prep + Cook Time: 60 minutes) Add lamb roast

to Ninja Foodi, add onion soup, beef broth, salt, and pepper Lock

lid and cook on HIGH pressure for 55 minutes Release pressure

naturally over 10 minutes. Serve and enjoy!

Nice Beef Fajitas

INGREDIENTS (4 Servings)

2 tablespoons butter ,2 bell pepper, sliced ,2 pounds beef, sliced ,2 tablespoons fajita seasoning ,2 onions, sliced

DIRECTIONS (Prep + Cook Time: 7 hour and 13 minutes)

Set your Ninja Foodi to Saute mode and add butter, onion, fajita seasoning, pepper, and beef. Saute for 3 minutes, Lock lid and set SLOW COOK mode, cook for 7 hours. Serve and enjoy!

Mushroom Hats Stuffed With Cheese

INGREDIENTS (3 Servings)

10 ounces mushroom hats ,2 ounces parmesan, grated ,½ teaspoon oregano, dried ,1-ounce fresh parsley, chopped

1-ounce cheddar cheese, grated ,2 tablespoons cream cheese ,½ teaspoon chili flakes

DIRECTIONS (Prep + Cook Time: 16 minutes) Mix together the chopped pars0ley, cream cheese, chili flakes, grated cheese, and dried oregano. Fill up the mushroom hats with the cheese mixture Place the mushroom hats in the rack. Lower the air fryer lid Cook the meat for 6 minutes at 400 F. Then check the

mushroom cooked or not if you want you can cook for 2-3 minutes

more. Serve hot and enjoy!

Mushroom And Bok Choy Health Bite

INGREDIENTS (3 Servings)

10 ounces bok choy, chopped ,1 tablespoon coconut oil ,5 ounces

white mushrooms, chopped ,1 teaspoon salt

DIRECTIONS (Prep + Cook Time: 14 minutes) Mix together

the mushrooms and bok choy. Add all the ingredients and mix them

well Sprinkle with coconut oil and salt. Make a shake to the

ingredients and place them into Ninja Foodi. Lower the air fryer lid.

Cook the side dish for 7 minutes at 400 F Stir generously. Serve

hot and enjoy!

Conclusion

Did you appreciate attempting these new as well as tasty dishes?

>Regrettably we have actually come to the end of this cookbook regarding making use of the amazing Ninja Foodi multi-cooker, which I actually hope you delighted in.

To boost your health and wellness we would like to recommend you to incorporate exercise as well as a vibrant lifestyle along with complying with these great dishes, so regarding emphasize the enhancements. we will certainly be back soon with an increasing number of interesting vegetarian dishes, a big hug, see you quickly.